# EVERYTHING YOU NEED TO KNOW ABOUT YOUR MENSTRUAL CYCLE AND FERTILITY

Written By:  Sam Hall

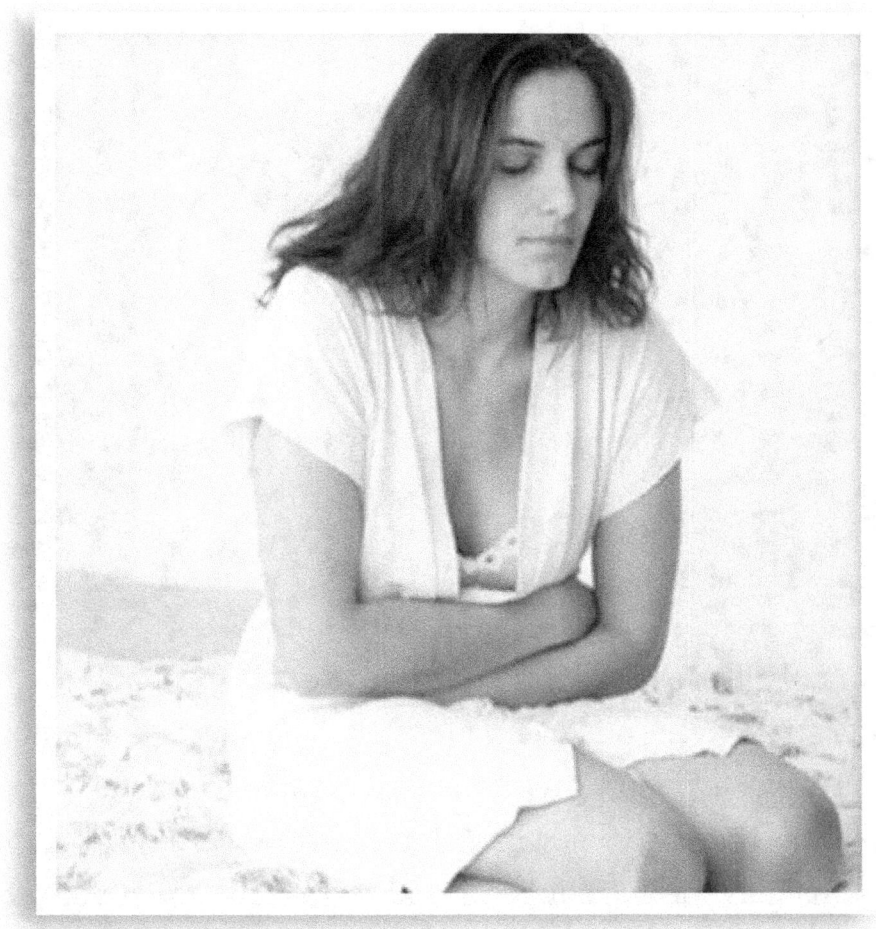

Women have special concerns when it comes to the "blessing" that is the female form. One of the most obvious of these is the monthly "time" that we all experience as our body prepares itself for the possibility of a healthy pregnancy. Even if you aren't sexually active, or you are on birth control, it's good to know all of the ins and outs of what's going on down there.

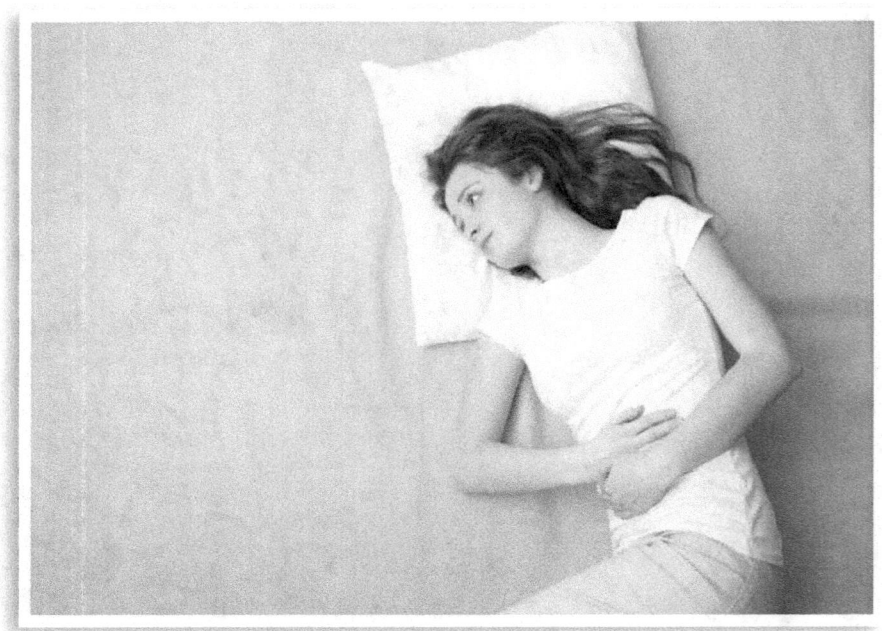

First of all, every woman experiences some form of the menstrual cycle, and every menstrual journey is different. You aren't ever going to fit the exact mold of "normal," because there is no normal.  However, there are certain truths that you can count on, and certain signs that you should look for and talk to your doctor about.

# THE BASICS

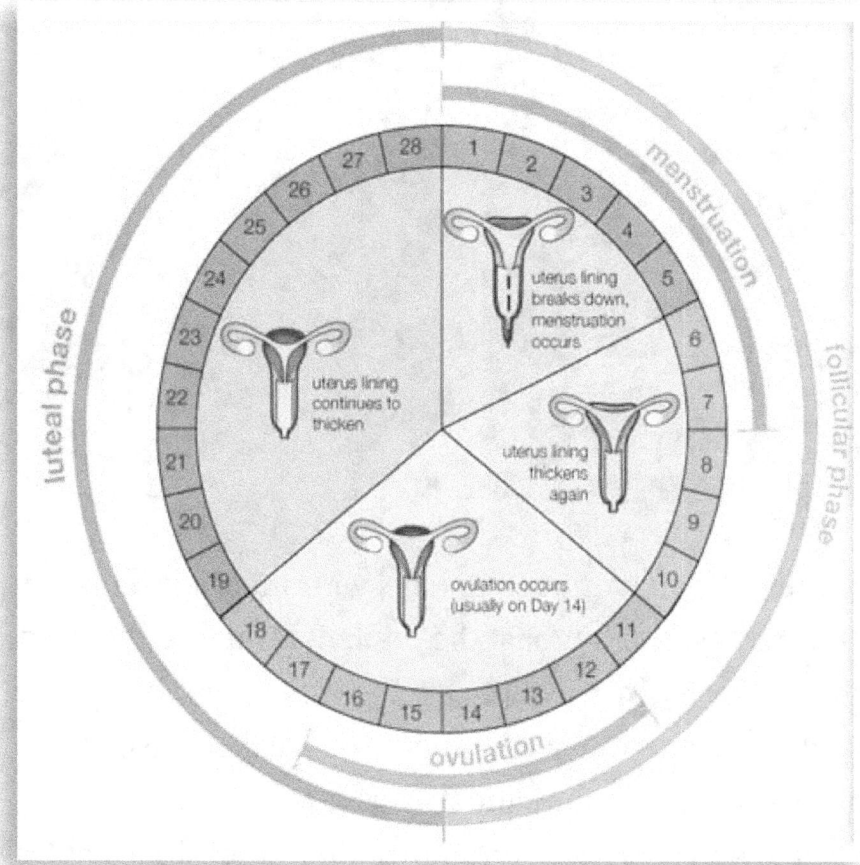

The menstrual cycle occurs roughly every 21-35 days in healthy women over puberty age who are not pregnant, or who don't have other concerns such as interruptions in their cycle due to certain methods of birth control. The full cycle is measured from the first day of one period to the first day of the next. Your cycles may be regular or irregular, but generally as your body matures you will find that there is more regularity.

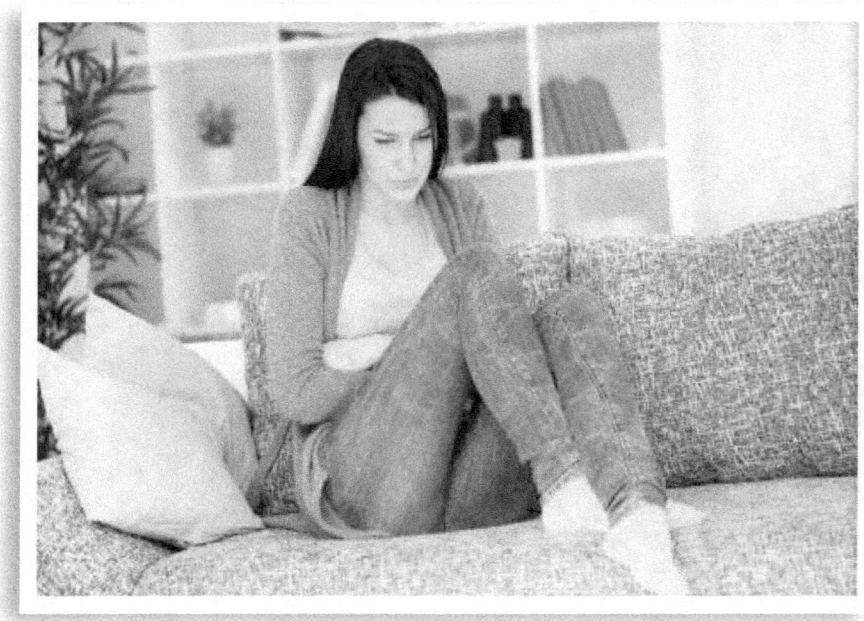

As you go about your normal life, your uterus is building a lining of tissue to support the implantation of a fertilized egg, so that it can grow into a fetus, and afterwards your sweet bundle of joy.  Each month, an egg is released from the ovaries (ovulation) and travels down the fallopian tubes toward the uterus.  At any point on this journey, the egg may be fertilized by an errant sperm, so make sure that you're keeping up on your birth control.

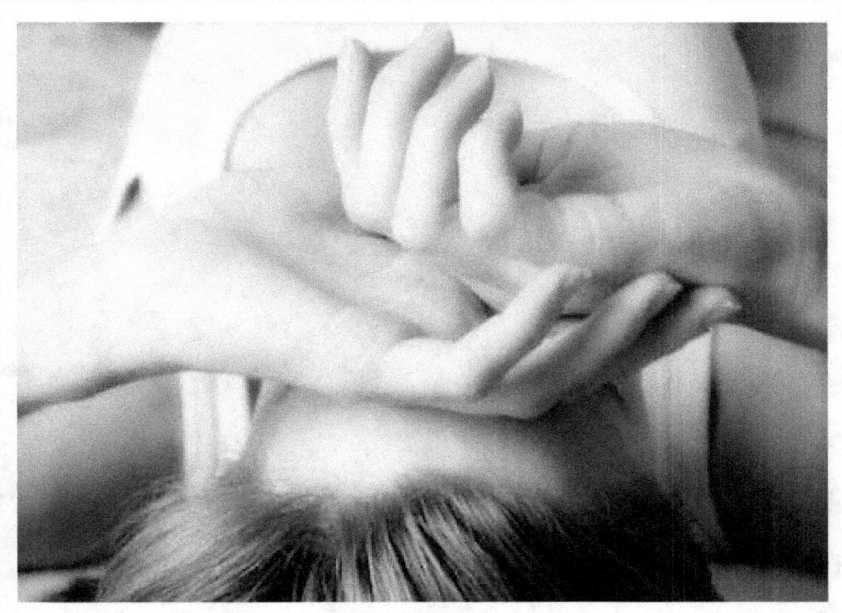

A fertilized egg will implant itself into the lining of the uterus, which then stays in place to nurture the rapidly multiplying clump of cells. This is why the earliest sign of pregnancy for many women is a missed or late period.

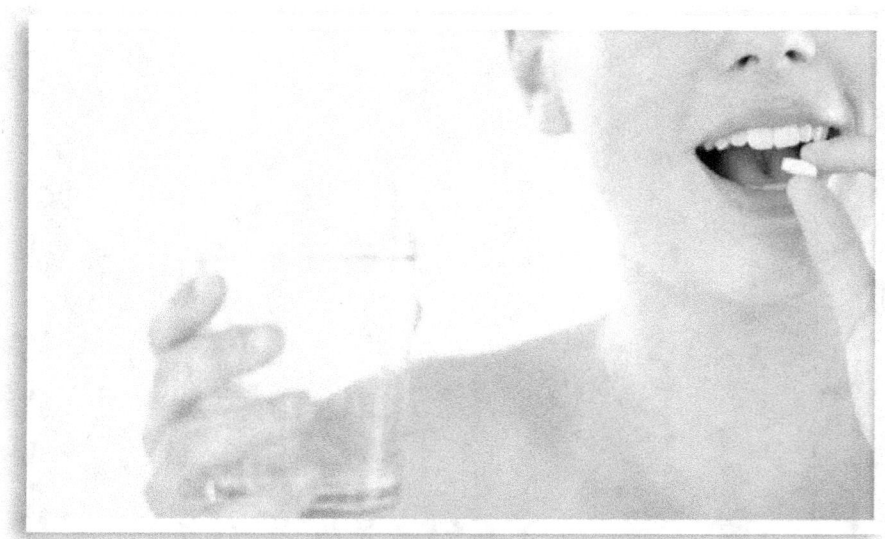

It's impossible to know until very close to your period whether or not you are pregnant for sure, which is why most OBGYN's will recommend that you stop drinking alcohol, smoking, and other harmful habits if you are planning to conceive a little one.  It's also a good idea to start taking vitamins ahead of time, especially folic acid to promote cardiovascular health.

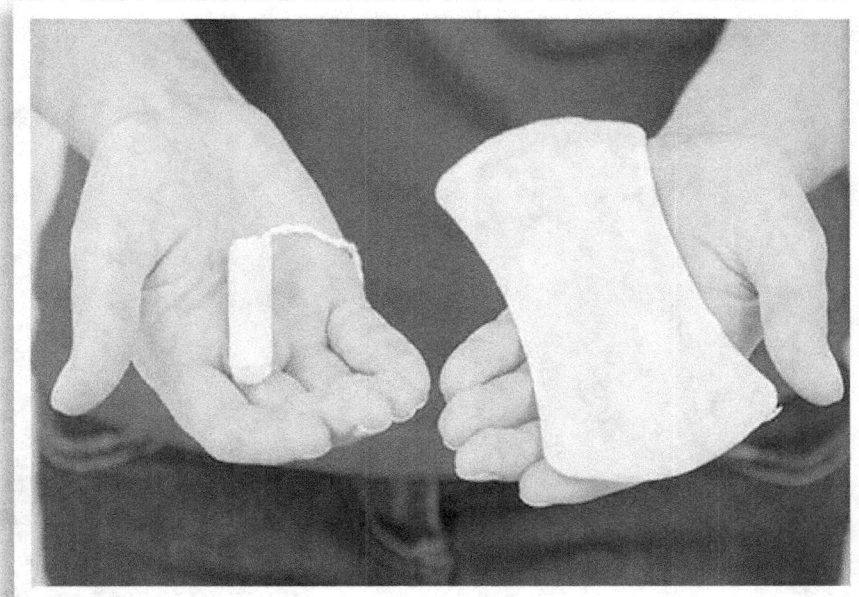

Your period occurs when the lining of your uterus is shed upon the completion of your eggs travel to the uterus without being fertilized. This can be a somewhat messy affair, so make sure to have tampons, pads, or a menstrual cup handy at all times, especially if you experience irregular cycles.

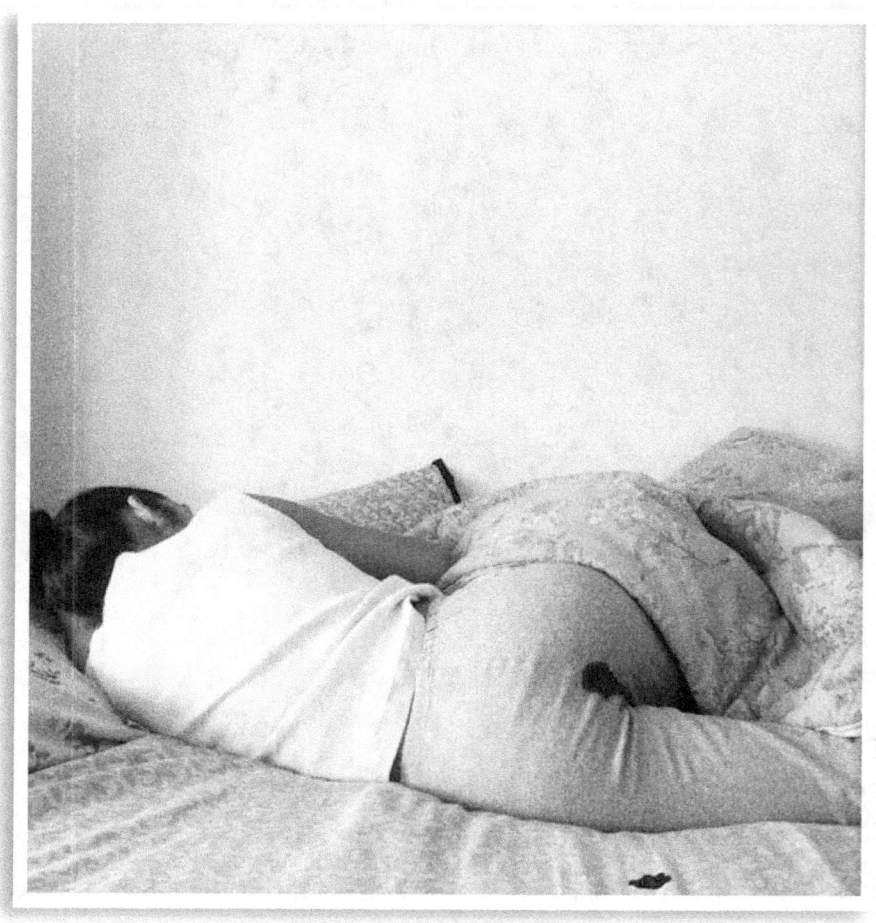

The length of time your period actually lasts can range anywhere from 2 to 10 days, and can be accompanied by a variety of other symptoms. The flow, as it's so charmingly called, may be heavy or light, and may taper off toward the end or stop abruptly. The discharge is often dark at the beginning of the period (especially for the first few cycles in young women), and may even appear brown.

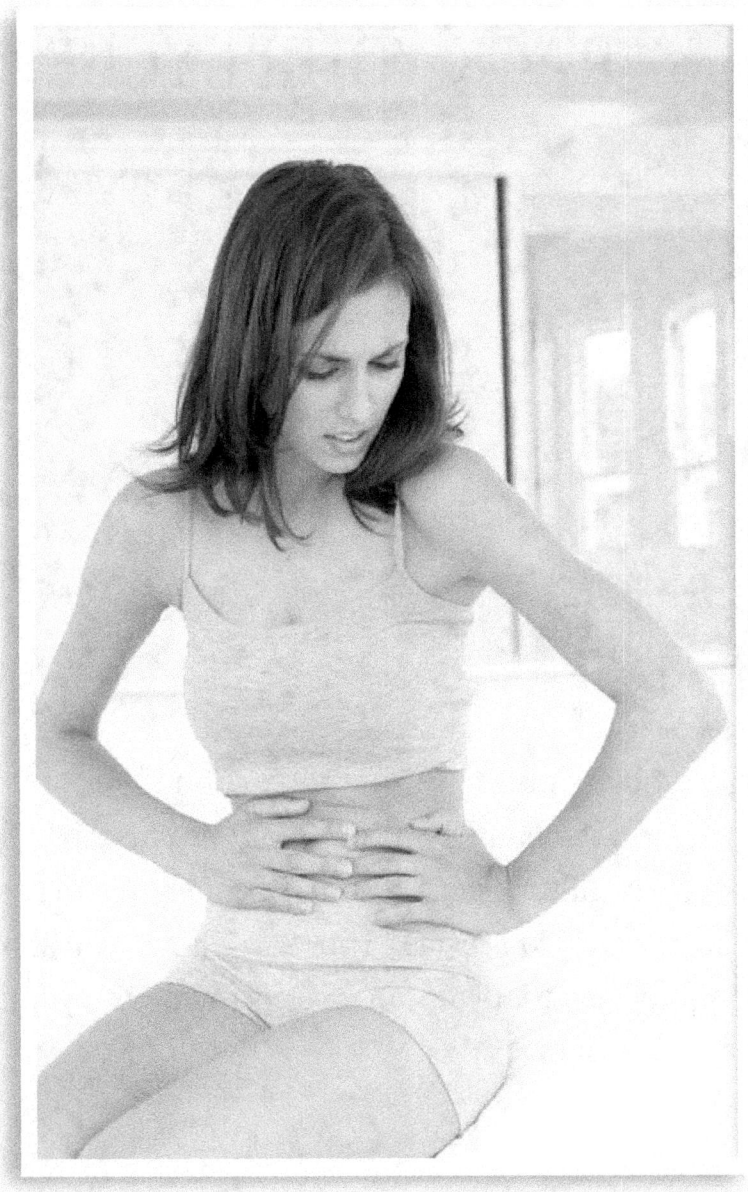

Many women find that they achieve a more regular cycle as the years go by, but if not don't despair. You'll figure out your body in time.

# TRACK YOUR CYCLE

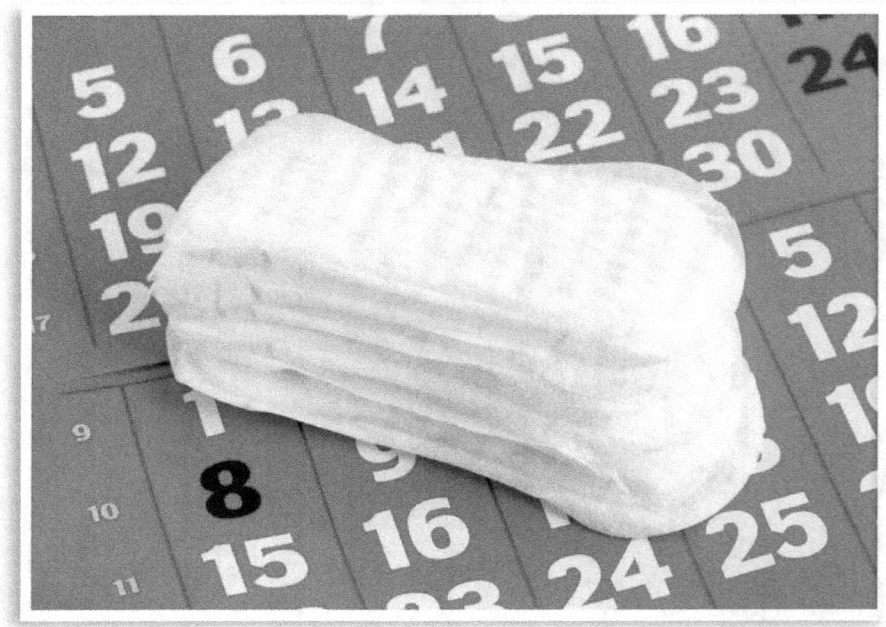

Whether you are new to this menstruation thing, or you are trying to get a handle on your body, or you are looking to conceive sometime very soon, it's a good idea to use a calendar to track your cycle.  These are things you should know offhand, so that you can discuss them with your doctor if necessary.

# LENGTH OF OVERALL CYCLE

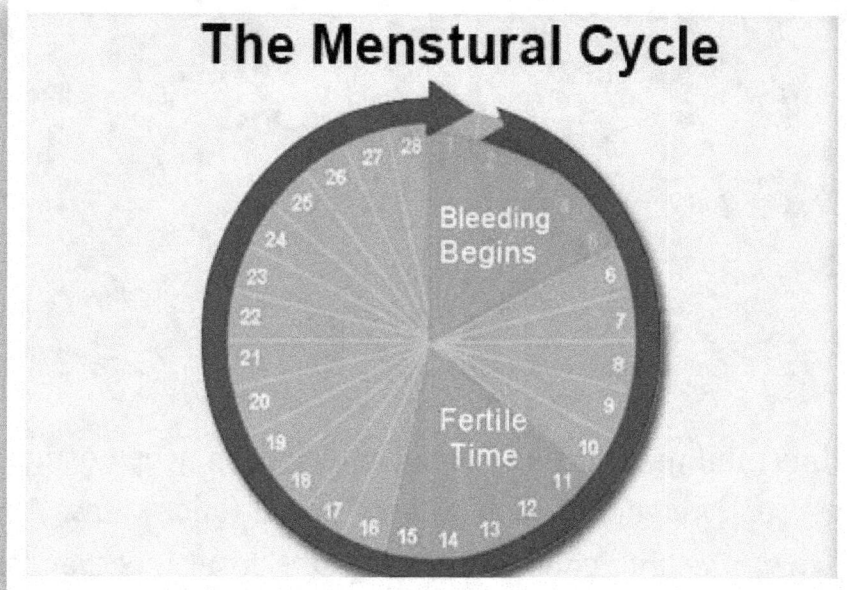

The length of your cycle starts on the first day of one period and ends the day before your next period. Knowing the length of your overall cycle will not only help you be prepared for when the flow starts, it will allow you to protect yourself from out of control PMS symptoms and time your points of ovulation if you are looking to conceive.

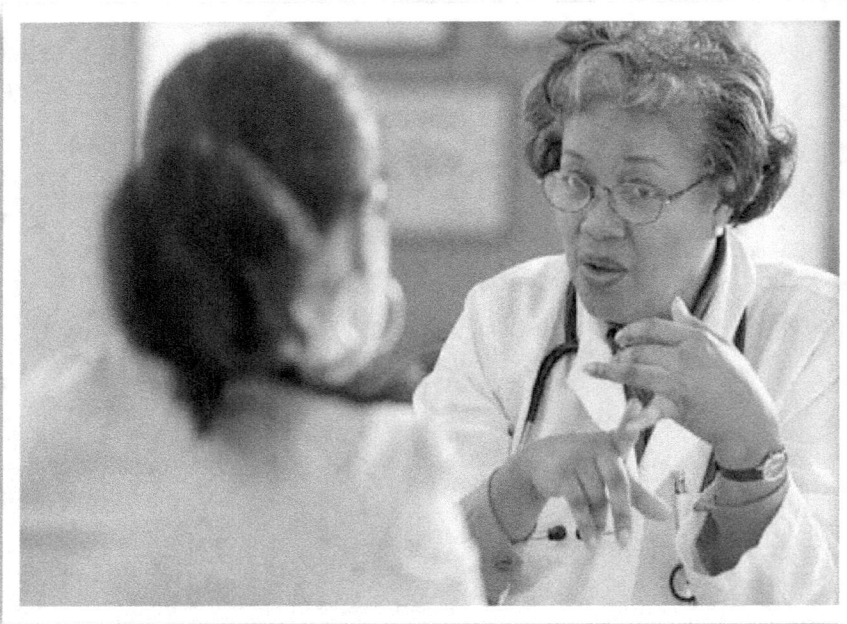

While minimal spotting between periods may be normal for you, it's a good idea to let your practitioner know. Also, if you notice that your periods happen closer together than 21 days and farther apart than 35 days, this might be cause for concern.

# LENGTH OF FLOW

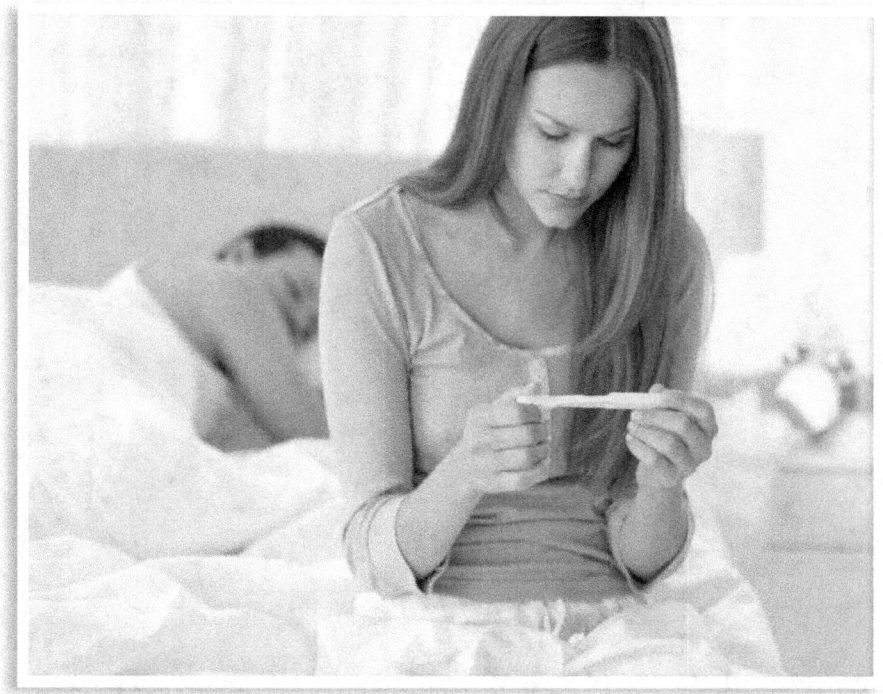

If you know about how many days your normal period lasts, you will have a better way to gauge if things have gone on too long. An extremely short period may be just that, or may be an indication of early pregnancy.

# HEAVINESS OF FLOW

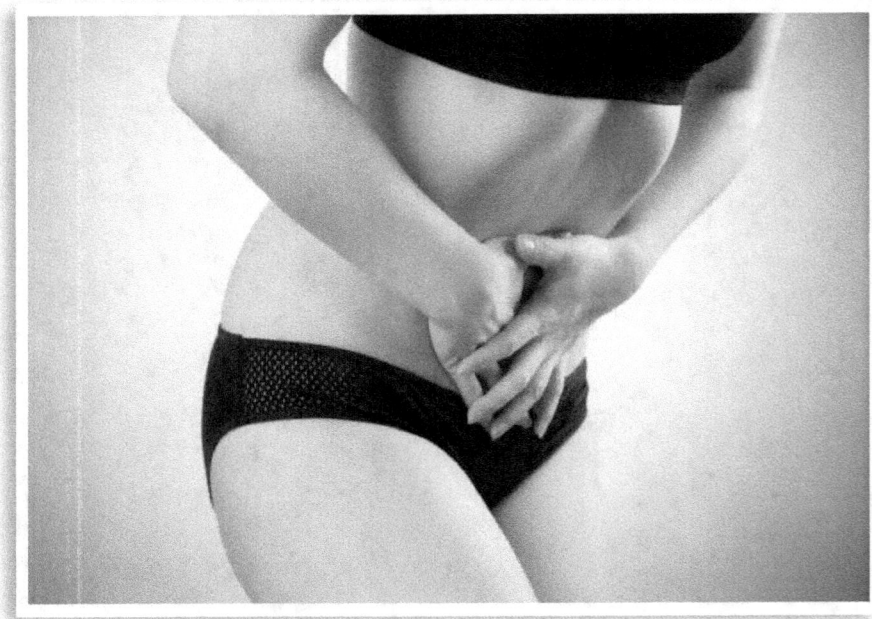

The heaviness of your flow will always be a concern for you, from the standpoint of what feminine products will be most effective. However, if your periods suddenly become much more heavy or light than they have been in the past, it's a good idea to have a doctor take a look.

# PMS

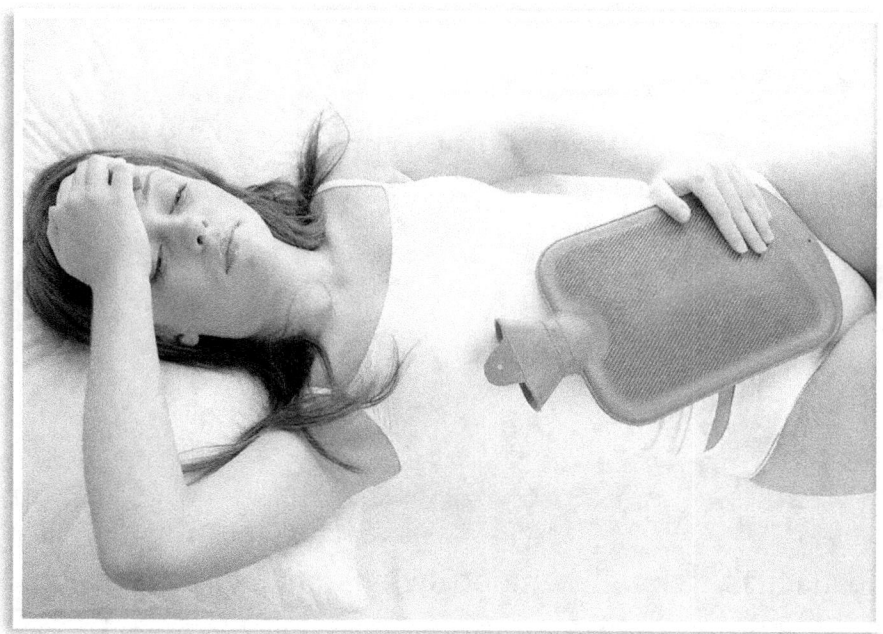

Pre-menstrual syndrome is a condition that occurs in the week or so leading up to your period when your hormones are out of whack and can give you any number of amazingly difficult symptoms that are seemingly unrelated to the impending river of blood that's hanging over your head.

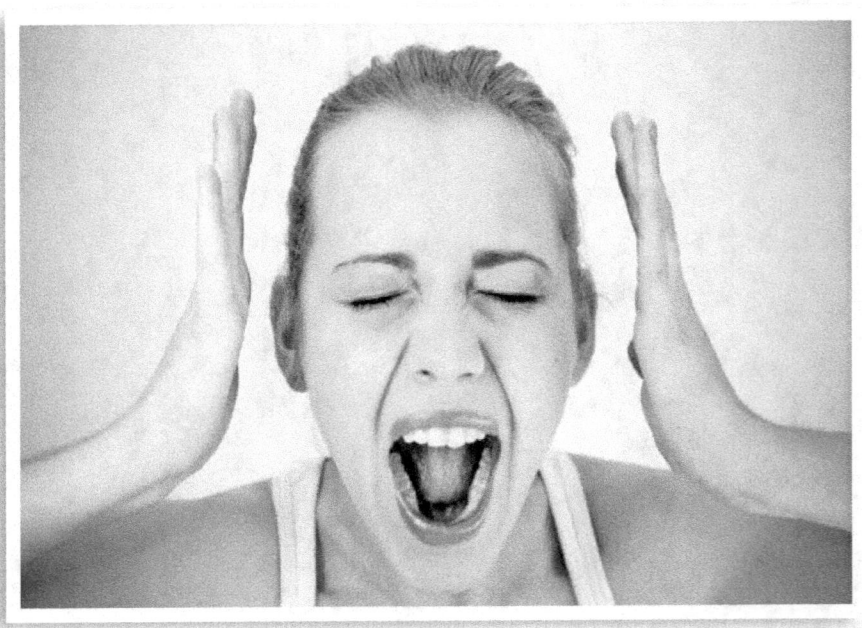

Headaches, irritability, mood swings, anxiety, depression, acne, bloating, constipation, diarrhea, upset stomach, appetite changes, tender breasts, and trouble sleeping are all part and parcel of the wonderful gift that is PMS in varying degrees. It's a good idea to know when these issues may crop up, which is yet another reason to keep a detailed menstrual calendar.

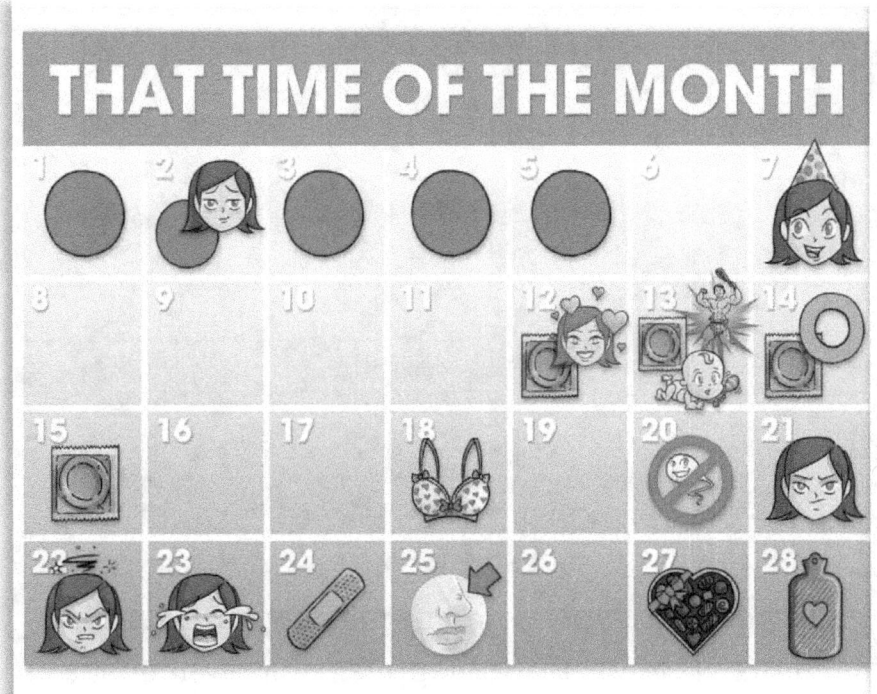

Welcome to womanhood! Now you've got a plethora of issues to deal with even leading up to Aunt Flow's visit, and a host of men who constantly joke about the uncontrollable roller coaster that you are on. If you notice that these symptoms are severe enough to interrupt your daily life, you'll want to mitigate them as best you can. It's a good idea to make note of recurring PMS symptoms on your menstrual calendar.

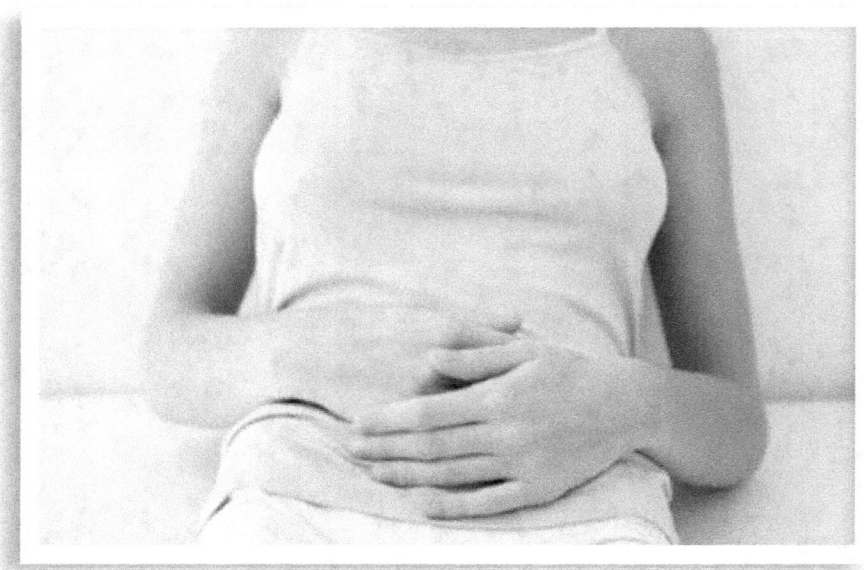

Headaches/muscle aches can be mitigated by over the counter medicines such as ibuprofen or acetaminophen. Make sure to follow the directions carefully to avoid liver damage. Other techniques for backaches include heating pads, warm baths, and a good old fashioned massage. Make sure you're staying hydrated to prevent headaches from getting too severe, and don't be afraid to lay down for a little nap when you feel the need.

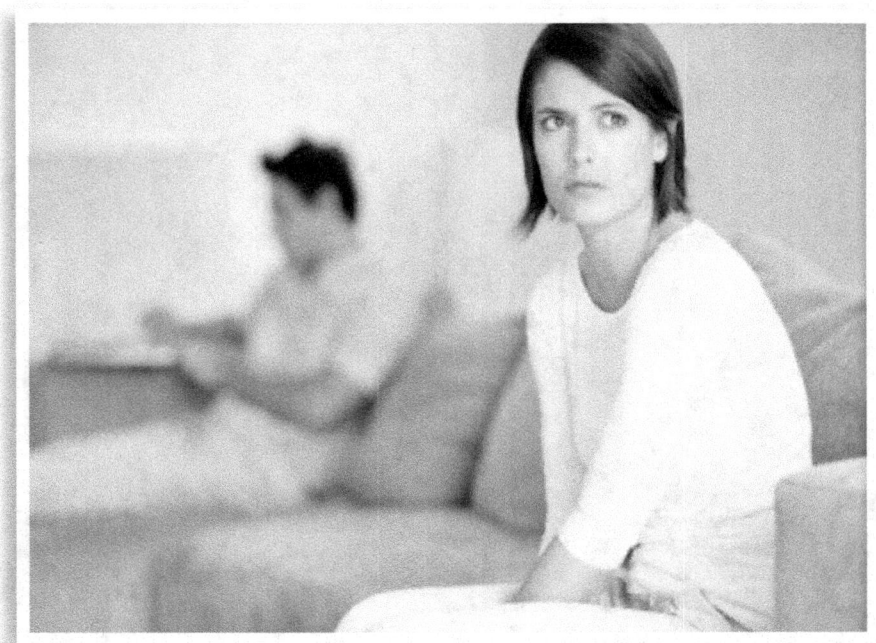

Mood issues such as irritability, mood swings, anxiety, and depression can be extremely difficult to deal with, especially when you're trying to get along in polite society. The best cure can be the knowledge that this is a symptom of your coming flow, and not all in your head. However, if you can't seem to shake the negativity through relaxation, journaling, and meditation techniques, it's worth the discussion with your OB.

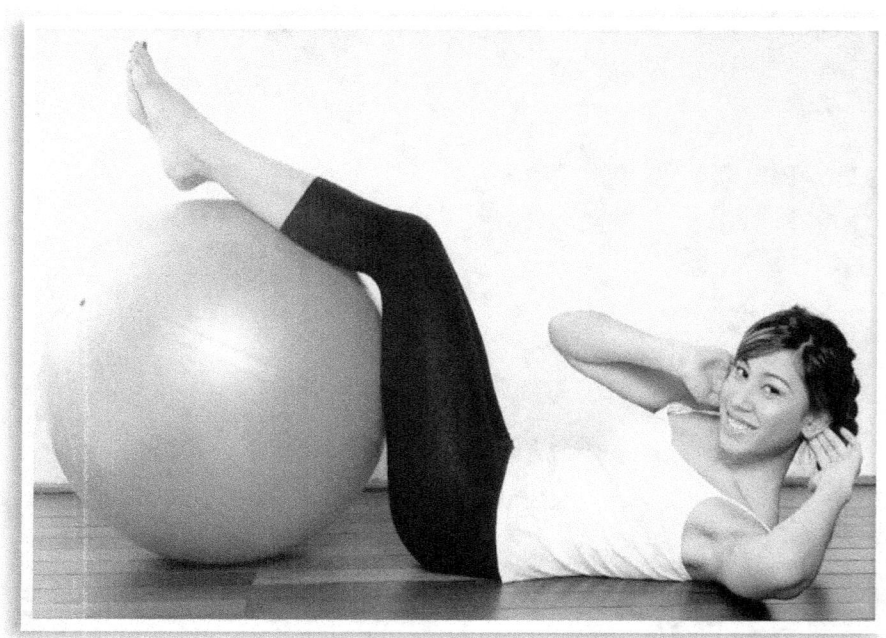

Lifestyle changes are often cited as the best cure for PMS, so if symptoms such as bloating, upset stomach, and other symptoms listed above become a recurring issue for you, it's time to really look at what you are doing to help your body cope with your cycle all through the month. Doctors recommend regular exercise, a balanced diet, and regular sleeping patterns as the number one way to find relief from recurring symptoms.

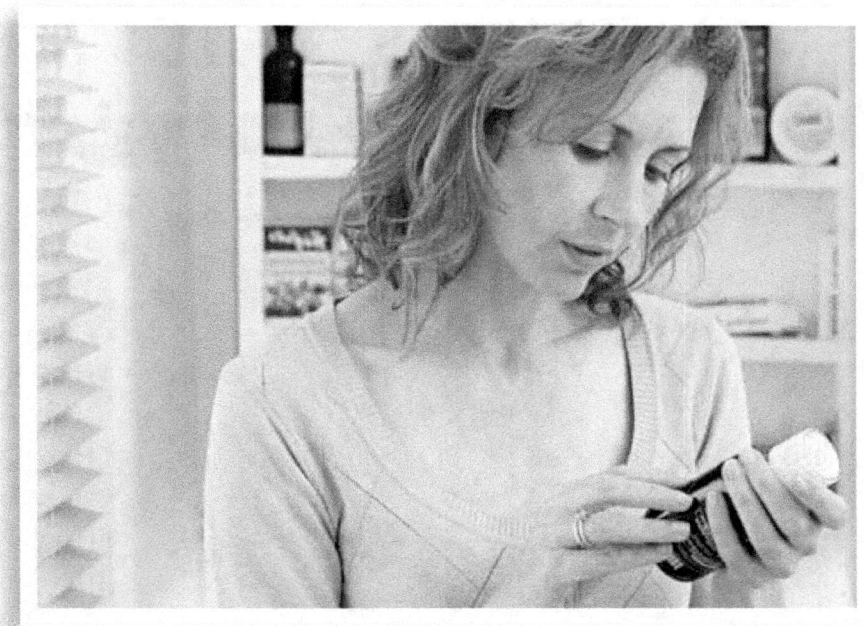

Medications are sometimes recommended by your doctor if all of the above mediating techniques are not enough, but there are possible side effects that you should be aware of. Make sure to read all of the labels, and realize that overuse of NSAID pain relievers can cause severe liver damage, especially if coupled with the use of alcohol.

# MENSTRUAL SYMPTOMS

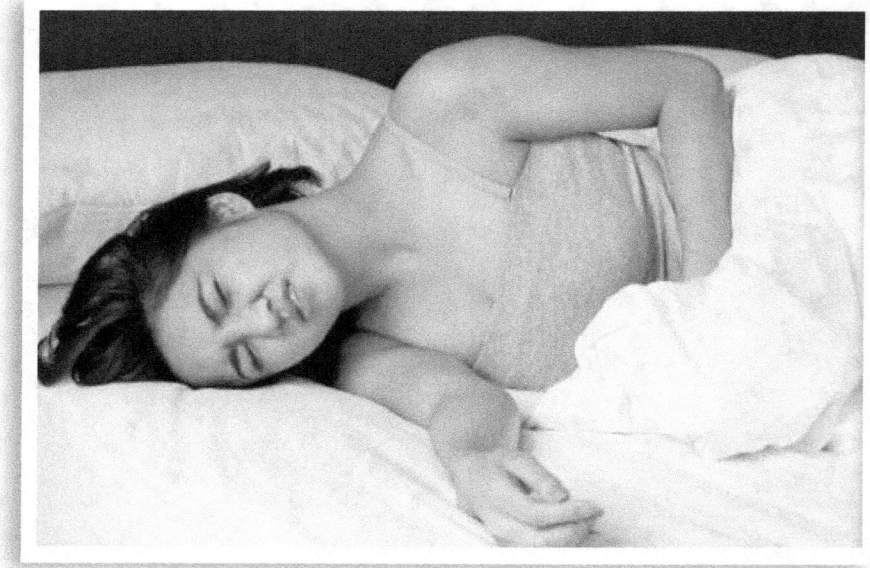

As if the actual blood flow was not enough to deal with, you may experience a myriad of symptoms during your period. The most common of these is abdominal cramping, which occurs when the muscles around your uterus contract in an effort to shed your uterine lining more efficiently. These can occur in the lower back as well as the lower abdominal muscles, and can be quite painful.

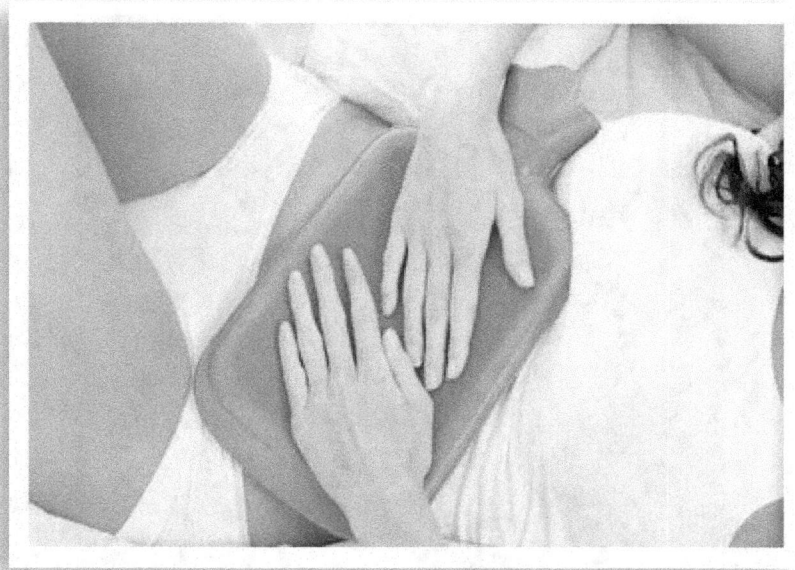

Deal with cramps the way that you would deal with any backache. Try mitigating with warm compresses, hot pads, and baths. Sometimes over the counter medications will do the trick. Whatever works for you, be sure to stay on top of it so that you don't go down for the count.

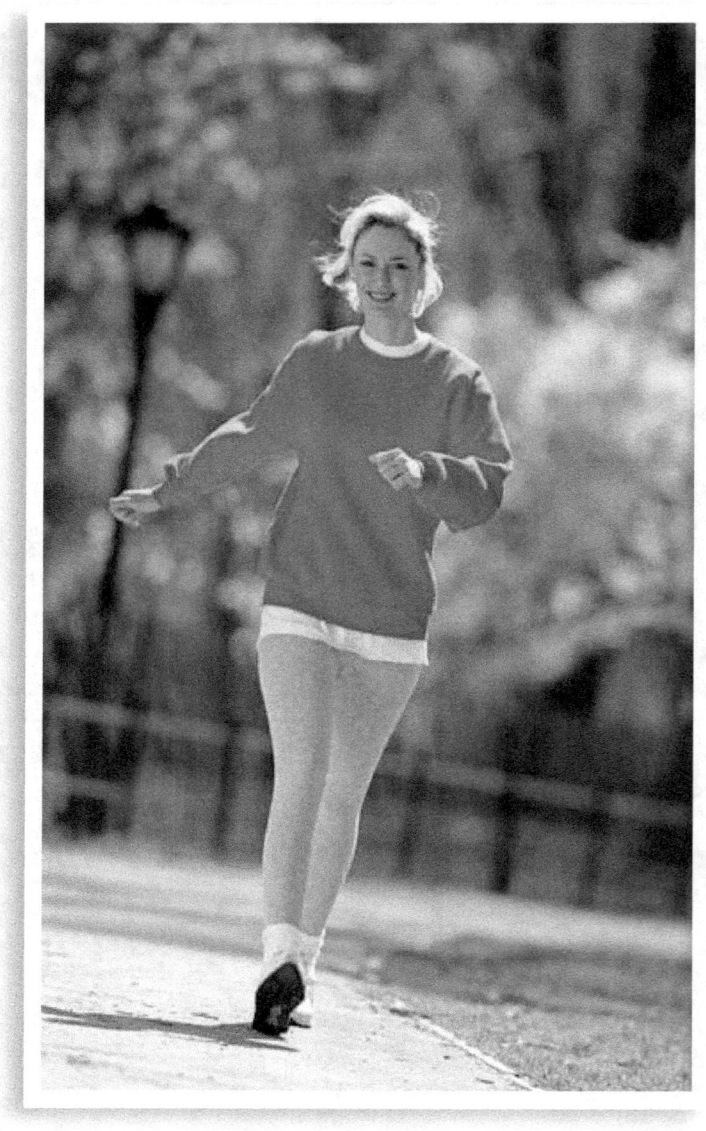

Sometimes the best cure for menstrual cramps is the one that is most counterintuitive. While you may want to curl up in a ball and cry, try to get your blood flowing through your muscles with a brisk walk around the block. The movement will be a great distraction at the very least, and may jump start you toward getting on with your day.

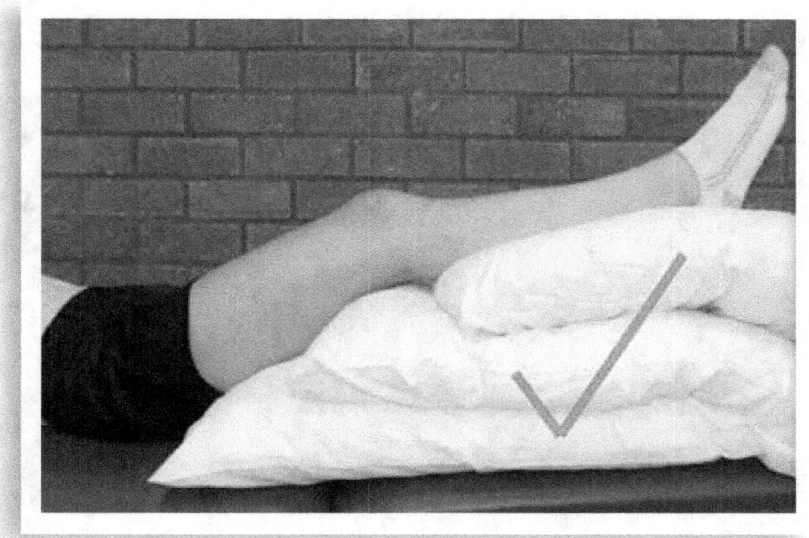

If you absolutely can't bring yourself to get up and move around, try elevating your legs when you lie down, and rotating your position periodically.

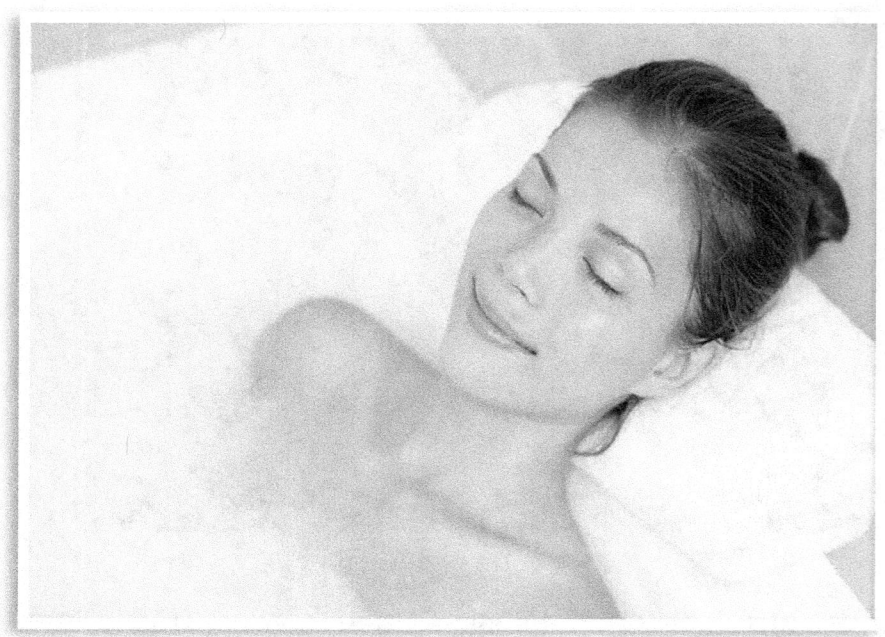

Vaginal pain when menstruating plagues many women, and can be made worse through the use of tampons. Try sanitary napkins or a menstrual cup if this applies to you. A heating pad may also increase your blood flow sufficiently to relieve pelvic pain. A warm bath can help with this, but avoid additives to the bath which can irritate sensitive skin.

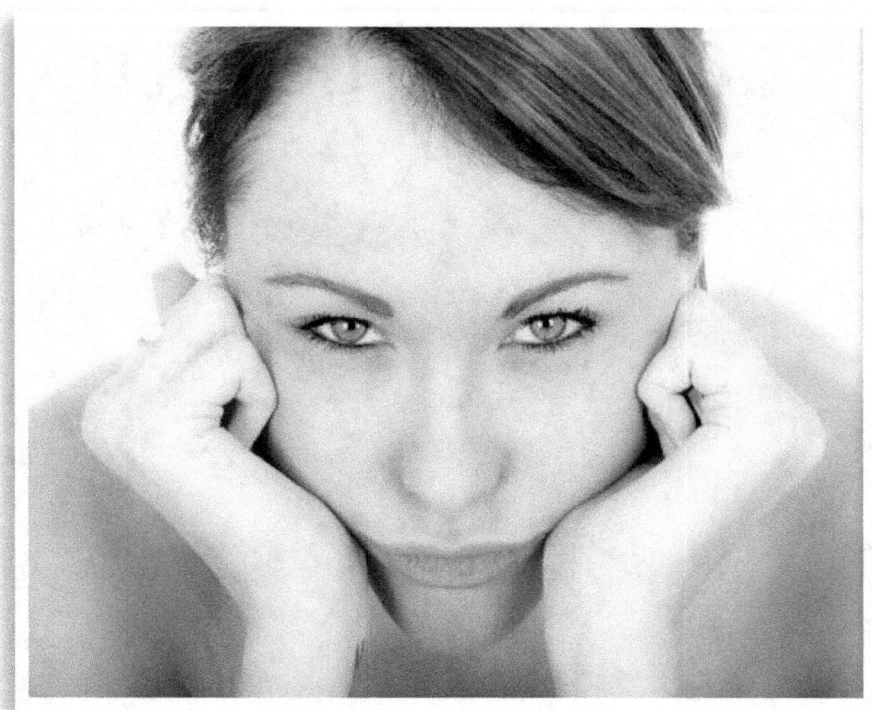

It's likely that any PMS symptoms, such as bloating and mood swings, that you experience before your period will carry over through the end of your period. Continue to do anything and everything that works for you.

# MANAGING BLOOD FLOW

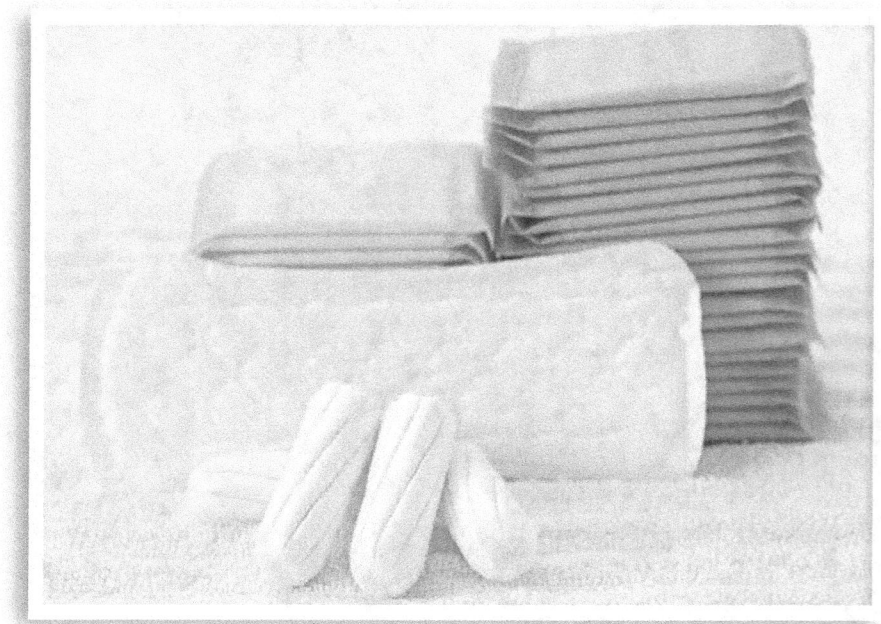

The shear number of products out there to help you manage your blood flow discreetly can be a bit overwhelming, and you may have to try a few different options to find out what works for you. Below are the most popular options and their benefits and drawbacks.

# SANITARY NAPKINS

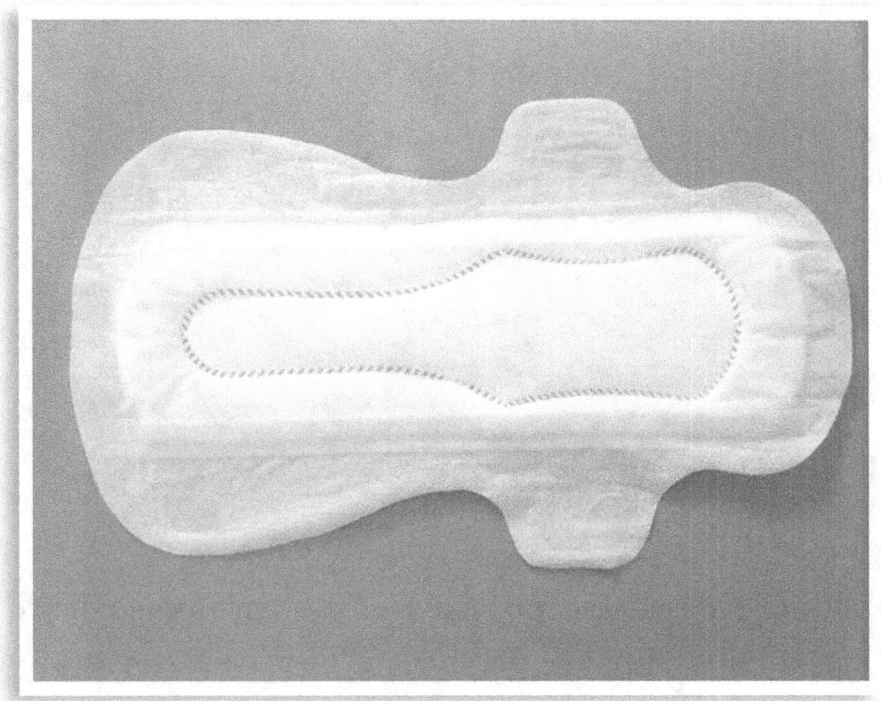

Sometimes called pads, these little guys sit in your underwear to catch the discharge as it leaves your vagina. These are best for women who experience any vaginal pain during menstruation, or who feel uncomfortable with the prospect of placing anything in their vagina.

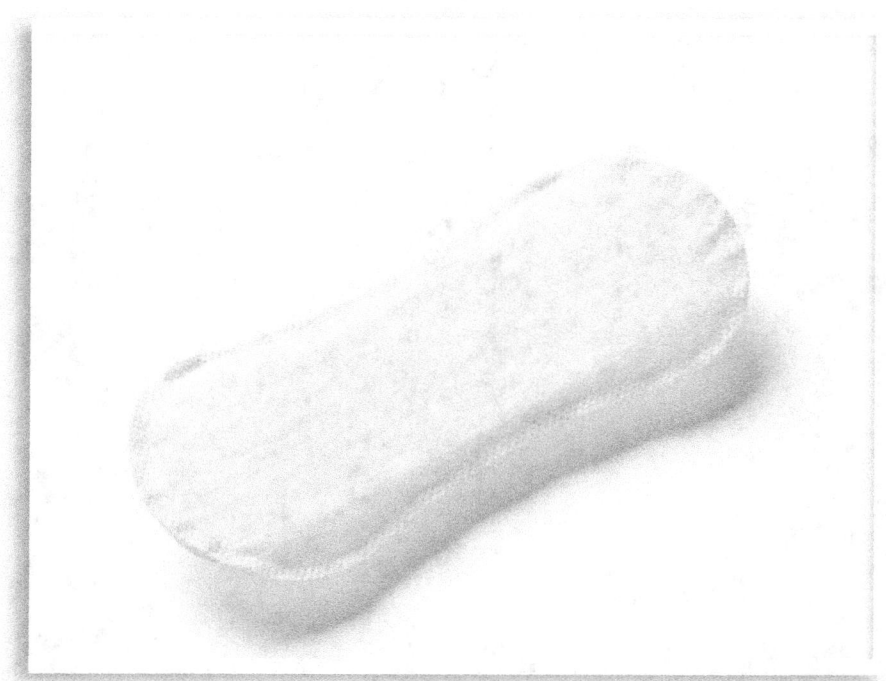

Pads are also the best alternative if you can't remember to change your tampon or empty your menstrual cup on a regular basis, as they have the lowest risk for infection.

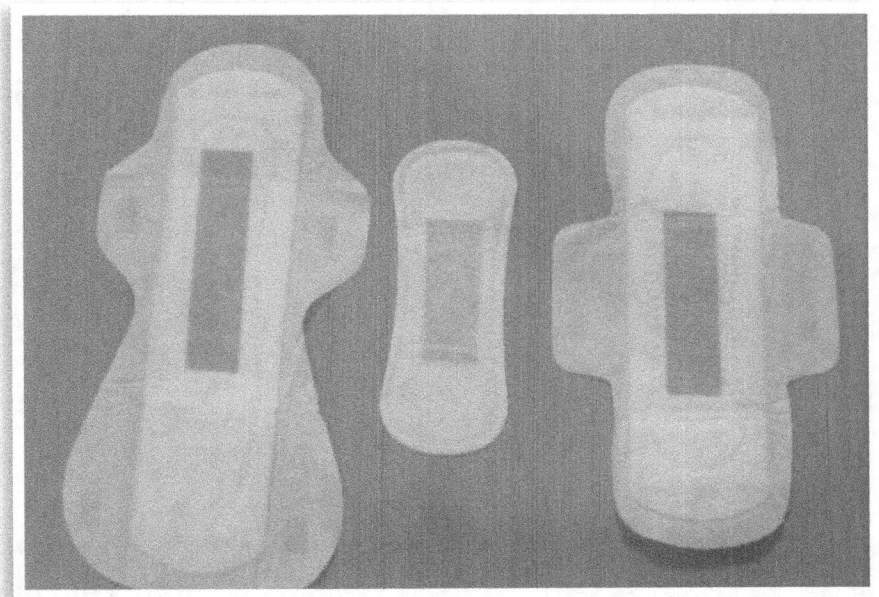

The main drawback to pads are that they are a bit messier than the alternatives. Active women may experience some overflow from the pad if it becomes dislocated from its optimal position. Some women experience discomfort from the lack of airflow that a pad can cause. Additionally, some feel that there may be an odor that comes from wearing pads for long periods of time, so they may actually have to be changed more often.

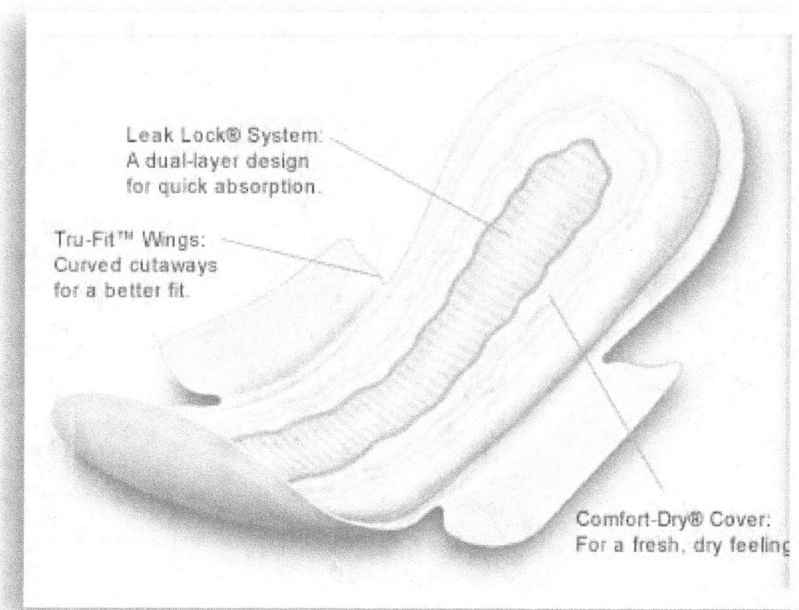

Leak Lock® System:
A dual-layer design
for quick absorption.

Tru-Fit™ Wings:
Curved cutaways
for a better fit.

Comfort-Dry® Cover:
For a fresh, dry feeling

As with anything that comes in contact with your lady bits, you're going to want to avoid heavily scented products that can irritate your skin. If you do notice skin irritation, immediately switch brands of pads and opt for something unscented and natural to help you out. Many women find that pads with wings are larger, but stay in place much more reliably.

# TAMPONS

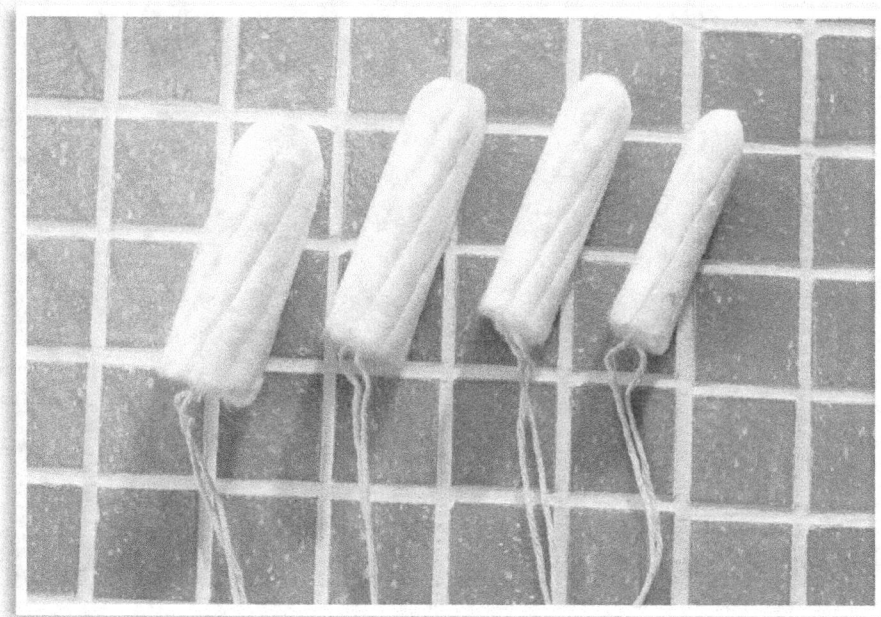

These little cotton buggers serve as a sort of plug to catch vaginal discharge before it leaves your body. Each one comes with a string attached for easy removal. These are by far the most popular choice for women who have had their periods for a long time.

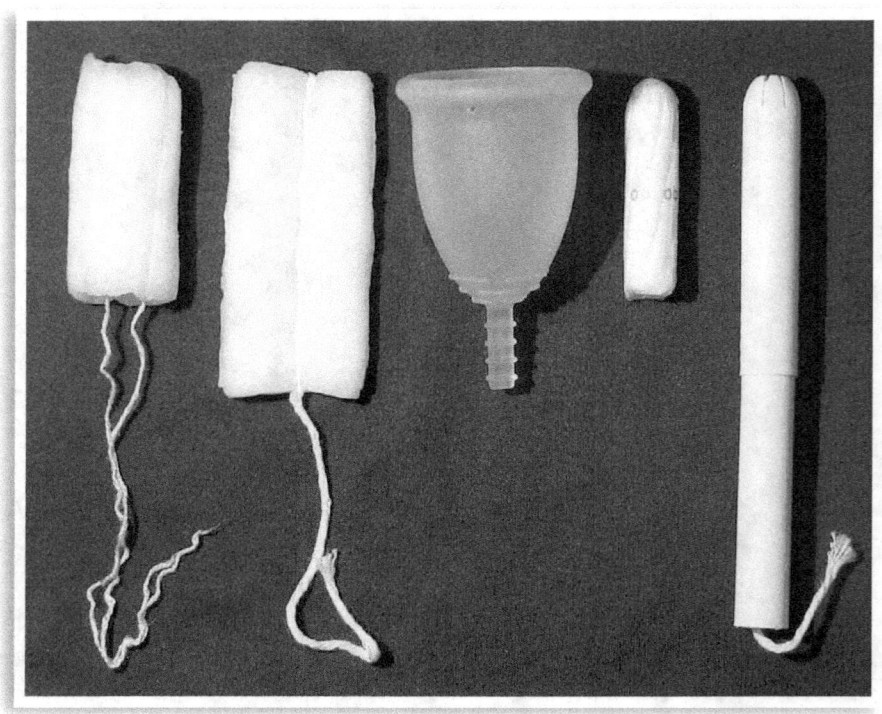

It is always wise to use the smallest tampon available that will handle your blood flow, and to change the tampon every four hours. This will reduce the risk of toxic shock syndrome, which is a very serious condition. If you notice that you begin running a fever while wearing tampons, or you experience vaginal discomfort, immediately remove the tampon. If the symptoms persist, seek medical advice.

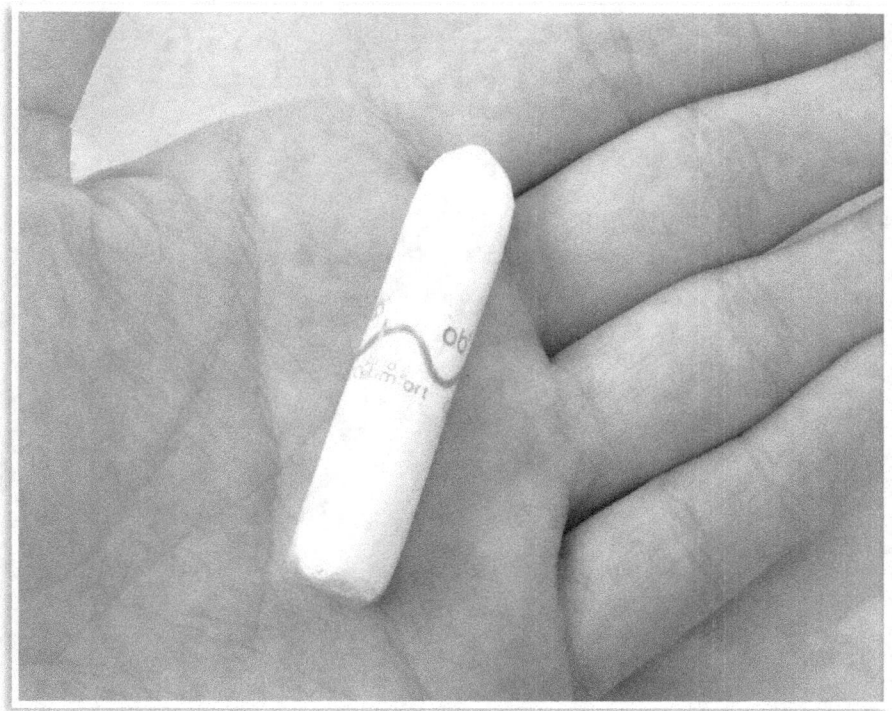

Vaginal discomfort with tampons can occur if you have a sensitivity to the components in the product, or the bleach that is used to finish the product. There are natural alternatives out there that are made for sensitive vaginas if you'd like to continue using tampons.

# MENSTRUAL CUP

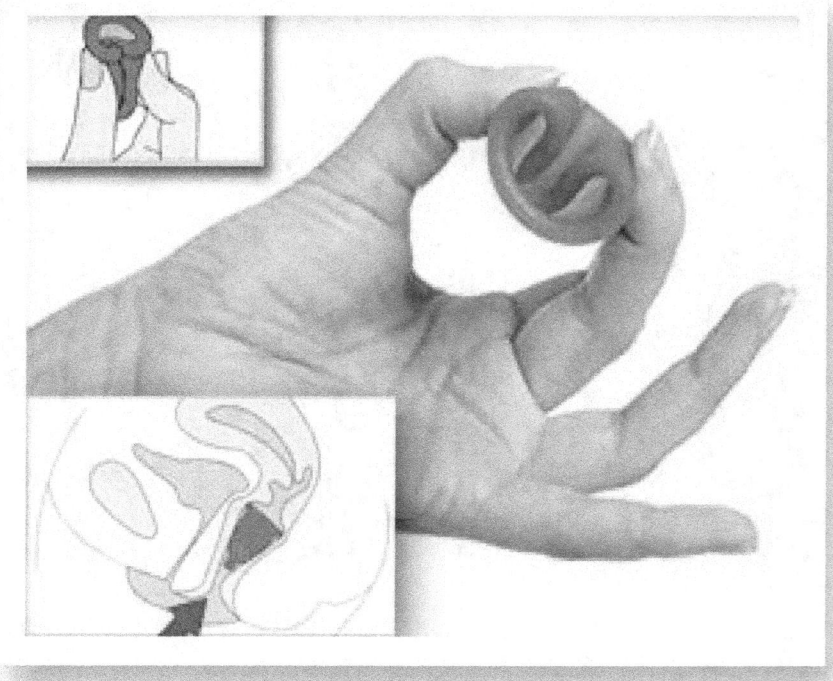

The menstrual cup is a relative newcomer onto the period scene, but some women swear they will never go back once they've tried it. A rubber cup is placed into the vaginal canal just below the cervix to catch your flow before it exits the body.

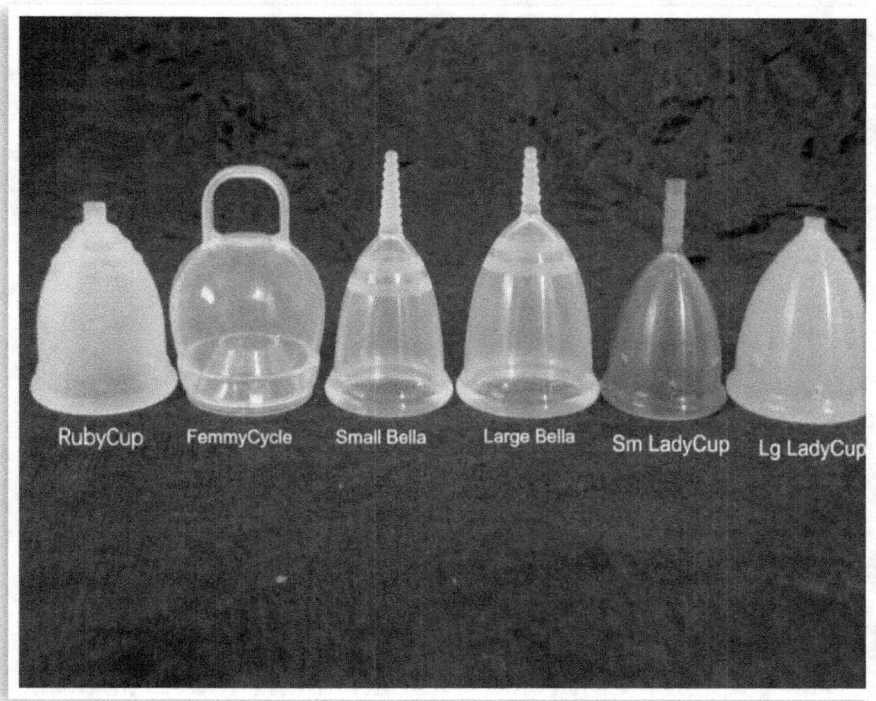

There are a few sizes of menstrual cup, and several brands. The size of cup you should order is determined by your age, sexual experience, and whether or not you have experienced vaginal birth.

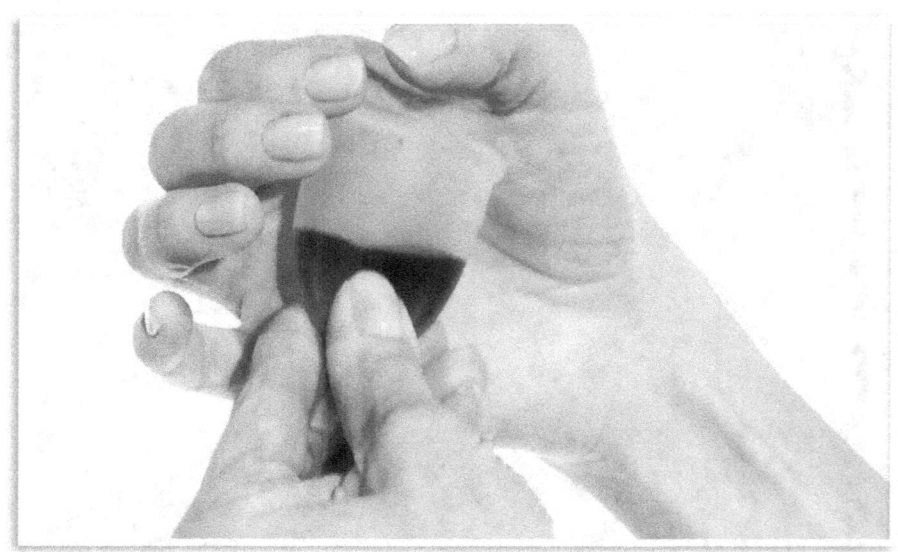

Women who are sensitive to tampons, but dislike using pads, swear by this method. It also reduces your risk of TSS as you must empty out the cup before it overflows... or have to purchase some new pants.

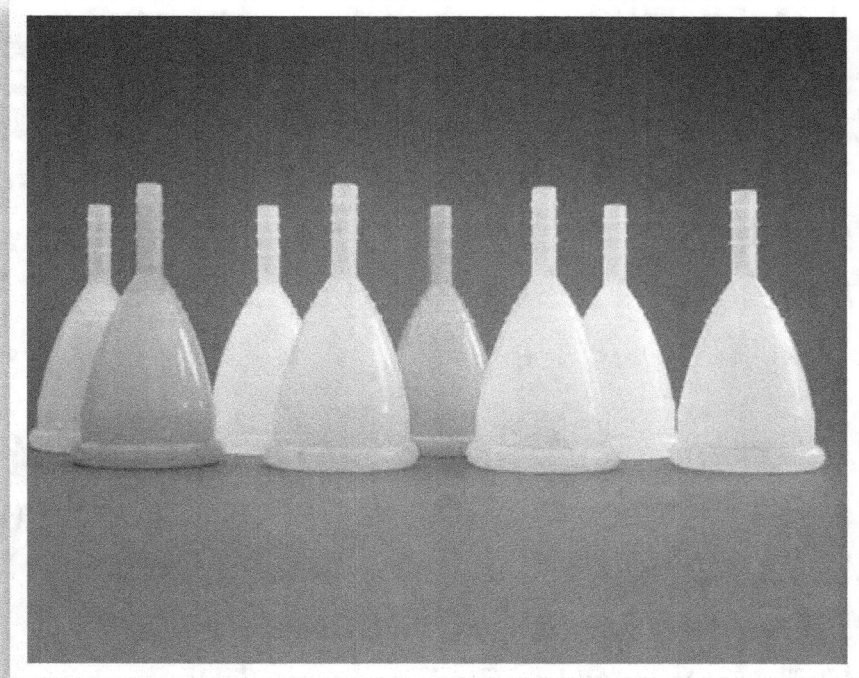

There's a cost benefit to using the menstrual cup as well. While there's a pretty hefty up front investment of $40 or so, the cups last an extremely long time if they're well taken care of and properly sanitized and stored. Most women find that this is a huge cost savings over purchasing pads and tampons for each cycle.

*Thank You!*

*We hope you enjoyed the book! All pictures and words were lovingly put together by experts who really love what they do! We really hope you learned something new today!*

*We would really appreciate it, if you could PLEASE take the time to let us know how we're doing by leaving a review on the Amazon website. We appreciate any comments you may have – what you enjoyed about the book, what additions you would have liked to have seen and what you would like to see in future publications.*

*Any comments will help understand better what you and your kids most enjoy and allows us to better provide exactly what you want!*

*Thought Junction Publishing*

# A NOTE FROM THE WRITER

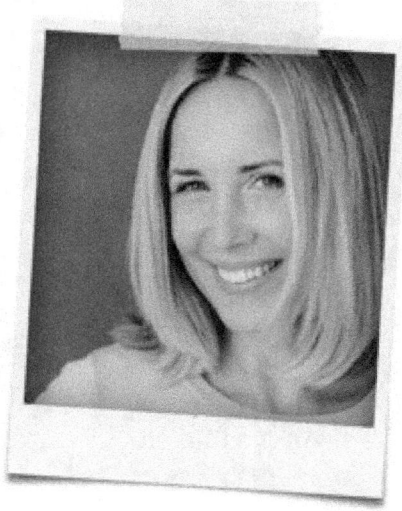

Sam's life revolves around her family, devoted mother of 3 - Noah (6), Oscar (3) and Poppy (11months) - she writes in a real way, aiming to answer the questions that other books don't cover, to fill in the blanks and inform parents and parents-to-be of the truth about raising children in the modern world.

Sam's writings emphasize that the readers are not alone - that there is a community of support available, and other people to talk to who can help, support and assist.

When she's not writing books, Sam is an advisor and avid blogger for Ideal Parent - http://ideal-parent.com - spreading support, care and advice across the web!

Join Sam on Ideal Parent and keep an eye out for her books - she's on a mission to help parents worldwide - join her and spread the word!

www.ingramcontent.com/pod-product-compliance
Lightning Source LLC
Chambersburg PA
CBHW061802280526
45787CB00003BA/1451